The Silver Solution to Women's Wellness

Using the NEW Structured Silver for All Areas of Female Health

Second Edition

Gordon Pedersen Ph.D., ND
Board Certified in Anti-Aging and Regenerative Medicine

About the Author

Gordon Pedersen is a Naturopathic Doctor (ND) with a Ph.D. from the Toxicology program at Utah State University. He also has Ph.D. degrees in Immunology and Biology. He is board-certified in anti-aging and regenerative medicine and also holds a Master's degree in Cardiac Rehabilitation and Wellness. He performed an internship with Jonas Salk, the American medical researcher noted for the discovery and development of the polio vaccine. He has formulated over 150 products, was a bronze medalist in the 2003 Utah Winter Games and is a best-selling author.

Gordon has spent countless hours reviewing silver information and is frequently called upon as the world's leading authority on silver as a health tool. He is a member and distinguished speaker for Special Operations Medical Association (SOMA) and has spoken with several national and international governmental organizations about silver. He has volunteered and personally funded efforts to bring silver's benefits into Africa's poorest communities with dramatic results including his published cure for malaria (10).

Gordon wrote this booklet to help as many women as possible enjoy improved personal health. He hopes that it will be helpful for women around the world, raising awareness of how silver provides new answers to age-old health questions.

Table of Contents

PART 1:
INTRODUCTION

On any given day, approximately one in four women will be suffering from some kind of vaginal problem. Yeast infections, staph infections and human papillomavirus (HPV) can cause problems that range from irritation to life threatening concerns.

The Need for Cleansing

The vaginal cavity is a warm, moist cavity, making it the ideal place for the growth of bacteria, yeast and viruses. Problems can result from poor hygiene, contamination, hormonal issues or genetics. The most common vaginal problems are bacterial vaginosis and yeast infections.

Disorders of the vaginal cavity are difficult to identify because the problems are not visible and the woman doesn't know of the existence of the problem until symptoms manifest themselves. Pain, itchiness, foul odor, redness, swelling, cramps or abnormal bleeding are often the first signs of a problem. All of these situations respond to vaginal cleansing, both as a preventive measure and as a treatment.

There is a remarkable new cleanse that utilizes new forms of Structured Silver. This cleanse addresses the cause of vaginal diseases. As such, many female health issues can be positively affected. Every woman could benefit from a silver vaginal cleanse at some point in her adult life.

The reason silver is so effective is that it has antibacterial, antiviral and antifungal qualities. Is it very difficult to identify the source of a vaginal problem because it could be bacterial, viral or fungal. Silver vaginal cleansing destroys all three of these sources of vaginal disease. It is the perfect vaginal cleanse. Silver can eliminate multiple sources of vaginal disease including antibiotic-resistant bacteria, STDs and yeast. And, most importantly, it can do so safely.

The need for improved vaginal hygiene is evident when you research the sexually transmitted diseases, yeast infections and occurrence of viral infections that cause cancer of the uterus and cervix. Silver destroys the cause of numerous vaginal diseases and has already become a woman's best friend when it comes to itching, odor, cramping and yeast infections.

What is This New Structured Silver?

Structured Silver liquid is a remarkably simple antimicrobial alkaline solution. It is composed of 0.001 percent pure metallic silver and 99.999 percent pure water.

That's it.

It is a clear liquid that looks, smells and tastes like water. That's because it is 99.999 percent water. Yet, it is changing the way we think of preventive medicine.

It is safe enough to self-administer and yet destroys the cause of the most dangerous diseases known to humanity. It is changing the way we prevent disease and defend ourselves against contagious diseases because it works even when we don't know what the disease is.

It destroys the cause of disease and does so with a greater spectrum of activity than any antibiotic, making it an alternative for antibiotics. Yet, unlike most pharmaceutical products, it has no side effects.

The silver particles have specific and unique characteristics, including a specific size, a specific electron configuration, a specific magnetic resonance, a specific pH, a specific magnetic signature and a specific structuring effect on the water molecules.

The resulting combination of silver and water has some very helpful properties. Some of these effects are best understood through the lens of physics as opposed to chemistry. Considering that most people view their health through the lens of biochemistry, the effectiveness of this new silver can catch people by surprise.

Specifically, the newest and most effective Structured Silver liquids can be identified by these characteristics:

- 10 ppm silver in water
- a mild alkaline pH (7.3 to 7.5 pH)
- molecular structuring (structured water)
- magnetic properties
- quality control that is vastly improved over old-style silvers

Silver technology has made huge improvements over the old-style colloidal silvers of 100 years ago. Structured Silver is today where penicillin was 80 years ago, but it won't have penicillin's problems and won't require a prescription. If you are using a silver liquid that is acidic, ionic or does not use structured water, you are not using the latest and most effective products.

Structured Silver comes in a liquid form and also as a gel. The gel form of silver contains a similar combination of silver and water, but has also been pH adjusted so that it is ideal for topical use. Although it contains more than just two ingredients, it has been made with maximum safety and purity in mind. Unlike many cosmetic products that contain carcinogens, pesticides, reproductive toxins and hormone disruptors, this new gel does not. With specific reference to the David Suzuki Foundation's "Dirty Dozen" list of substances to avoid in cosmetic products (1), Structured Silver gel does not contain:

- BHA or BHT (preservatives that may cause cancer & endocrine disruption)
- Coal tar dyes; p-phenylenediamine (artificial colors with heavy metals and cancer-causing potential)

- DEA, MEA and TEA (eg. triethanolamine)
- Bibutyl phthalate
- Formaldehydes
- Parabens
- Parfum
- PEGs (eg. polyethylene glycol)
- Petroatum
- Siloxanes
- Sodium laureth sulfate
- Triclosan

If you are using an unstructured silver gel that contains parfum, TEA or other substances listed above, you are NOT using the latest, best and safest products.

In summary, Silver is an unusual combination of silver and water that safely kills pathogens. It comes in a newly perfected structured form that offers outstanding benefits without side effects or harmful chemicals. It might save your life or the lives of people you love.

Silver Through History

Ancient Greeks used silver vessels for water purification. American pioneers trekking westward used it to keep their water safe and prevent dysentery, colds and flu. They also put silver dollars in their milk containers and wooden water casks to slow bacterial growth. Settlers in the Australian outback suspended silverware in their water tanks to retard spoilage. People in India still wrap some food and candies in a thin silver foil to prevent spoilage, which is then literally consumed along with the food.

Medicinal silver compounds were developed in the late 1800s and there was widespread use of silver compounds and colloids (small particles dispersed in water) prior to 1930. By 1940 there were approximately 48 different silver compounds marketed and used to treat virtually every infectious disease. These were available in oral, injectable and topical forms. They carried such names as: Albargin, Novargan, Proganol and Silvol. (2)

Since 1973, silver has been shown to have topical activity against 22 bacterial species (643 isolates) including gram positive and gram negative bacteria. (3) Ongoing research into the effect and properties of silver continues around the world.

Currently, silver water purification filters are used by organizations that include international airliners and NASA. Increasing numbers of Americans use silver in their fabrics, appliances and home water filters. Electrical ionization units are being used in swimming pools to help sanitize the water without the harsh effects of chlorine. Silver is also found in many applications within our hospitals, from needles to bandages to disinfectants for newborn babies' eyes. (4)

Silver has been used to treat burns and heal wounds for decades. Wounds heal faster and with less scarring when bacteria, viruses and yeast cannot contaminate the wound. Burn victims report a reduction in pain when silver liquid or gel is applied to the wound. Because silver can be applied in an open wound it can assist in disinfection and help stimulate the healing factors of the immune system. This is true for vaginal infections and internal bleeding in the uterus or cervix as well.

New advances with silver continue to be made in the pursuit of maximum effectiveness and safety. In just the past two or three years, brand new ways of structuring silver molecules into water have been developed that show significantly improved results when compared with earlier silver products. This is an emerging field in terms of public familiarity.

For women seeking new ways of controlling vaginal infections or other pathogen-caused problems, this is very good news.

Structured Silver is New – Critical Differentiations

This brings us to a critical point: Structured Silver is not the same as other silver products. Even other products that contain silver and water are not the same as Structured Silver.

One thousand years ago, people used primitive forms of silver and received mild antimicrobial benefits.

One hundred years ago, people used primitive colloidal and ionic silver products and received good antimicrobial benefits, but also suffered side effects like argyria. Argyria is a discoloration of the skin towards a bluish grey, but it is rare and non life-threatening. Argyria can occur with concentrated silvers (very high ppm, such as 50,000 ppm) and impure silver compounds (eg. silver salts) that precipitate within the body. Argyria cannot happen with Structured Silver when it is taken as suggested.

Ten years ago, people used more advanced silver solutions and gels and received excellent antimicrobial benefits and vastly improved safety standards.

Today, people have access to Structured Silver products that even outperform last decade's products. The new silvers are safer and more effective. When compared with last decade's top products at top U.S. laboratories and in clinical usage, today's Structured Silver shows significantly improved performance against pathogens and reduced healing times – as much as 40 percent faster.

Our ability to access silver's benefits have moved from primitive to good over the centuries, with new levels of excellence available now that are even better than last decade's best. Just as computers have developed at a rapid pace, so have silvers. A computer from twenty-five or even ten years ago was a good tool at the time, but how many people choose an old computer when faced with a design, communication, programming or entertainment need? Ten years old may be good, but it is no longer the best. As it is with computers, cameras and smart phones, so it is with silvers.

When choosing your silver products, be mindful of what you seek. You might not be able to see the differences with the naked eye, but they are real and can impact your health. If you were five or six micrometers tall, the differences between silver products would be as obvious as the differences between a horse and a cow. Yet, since you are likely closer to five or six feet tall, the differences between Structured Silver and other substances are invisible without closer inspection. In short, you do not need to use your grandma's silver. Just as horses and cows are similar yet critically different, old-fashioned silver products and Structured Silver are similar but critically different from one another.

With clarity on this point, a new health vector emerges. Without clarity, today's new silver products are incorrectly called 'snake oil' or worse, due to confusion with older technologies.

Unfortunately, many of today's medical experts remain ignorant of the interrelationship between physics, energy, healing and silver. When questioned about silver, many experts still respond in terms of biochemistry, which is a decades-old approach suitable for decades-old silvers that worked through biochemistry. However, the biochemical paradigm is insufficient for understanding and applying today's silvers, which are built with biophysics in mind. This is a huge shortcoming of today's medical field. A few doctors are making use of the latest silver technologies, but many more doctors still think in an obsolete paradigm.

Beyond Just Chemistry

As methods of using silver have advanced over the centuries, the primary focus has been on chemistry. Whether dealing with basic metallurgy or finding ways to access silver within a liquid, the questions have generally centered around, "What are the ingredients?" and "What size are the particles?" These questions

11

led us from using silver coins in our water supplies (the root of today's odd practice of throwing coins into public fountains) to basic colloidal silver products, ionic silver liquids and even recent hydrosols. These advances led humanity from primitive access of silver to a much better form.

However, the progress does not stop with chemistry. Newer forms of silver also use physics to further improve their applications. In addition to the questions of ingredients and size, leaders in the field are now also asking, "How does biophysics apply?"

For instance, did you know that silver is the best conductor of energy in the entire periodic table of elements, yet most of today's silver products do not take advantage of this? Many of today's popular silver products also do not take advantage of recent breakthroughs in magnetics that profoundly affect molecular structure, the characteristics of water and ultimately the ability of an end-product to defeat pathogens.

Summarized, by the year 2013 there are several silver products on the market with excellent chemistry, but very few with equally excellent physics. The difference in performance is clear in lab results and clinical healing times, but many people are not yet accustomed to thinking in terms of biophysics and thus find the differences confusing.

If you are new to the term "biophysics", I suggest taking a few minutes to do an online search for the topic. It will prove most illuminating. Very briefly, biophysics strives to address biological questions while using tools and principles from physics. This includes magnetism, wavelengths (including x-rays and MRI) and energy. Biophysics is already used in hospitals throughout North America, yet most people are still more accustomed to thinking of health within the biochemistry model that was dominantly explored and taught throughout the 20th century.

What Does Structured Silver Do?

Structured Silver kills germs. These germs may be living in the pores (causing acne), in the vagina (causing a vaginal infection), in an eye (causing pinkeye), in the digestive tract (causing gas or a serious health problem), in a wound (obstructing healing or causing scarring), around a piercing (causing infection), on the cuticles (causing inflamed hangnails), on the lips (causing cold sores), in the bladder (causing bladder infection), on the toenails (causing odor or unsightly infections), etc. Regardless of where they are growing, the problem is the same: germs are growing and disrupting your health.

If you can name an affected spot in or on your body and you can get silver into contact with germs that a growing there, that is where silver can help you. If you keep silver in contact with the germs for six minutes, these germs will no longer be able to cause you health problems.

Simply by killing germs, an amazing list of health problems can be helped or avoided.

Which Germs?

Structured Silver has been shown to be effective with several categories of pathogens. In contrast to conventional antibiotics that typically have a limited spectrum of activity (they only kill a few specific germs), this is unexpected and exciting.

Summarized, Structured Silver is a broad-spectrum antimicrobial that:
- destroys pathogenic bacteria
- inhibits viral replication
- destroys many fungi, yeasts and protozoa
- destroys the malaria parasite (10)

Structured Silver even kills antibiotic-resistant strains of bacteria such as MRSA. Antibiotic resistance is a major problem facing hospitals and homes around the world, as pathogenic bacteria no longer respond to antibiotics such as penicillin, methicillin, vancomycin and so on. Do an online news search at http://news.google.com for "MRSA" or "superbugs" and you will see how serious the problem is. Some bacterial infections no longer respond to any drugs and problem is getting worse. However, due to the fact that Structured Silver kills bacteria differently than traditional antibiotics, it kills resistant and non-resistant bacteria alike. This paragraph could easily be expanded into a book of its own, but the simple and relevant fact is this: Structured Silver eliminates pathogenic bacteria, including drug-resistant strains.

Despite this incredible ability to kill pathogens, Structured Silver is safe enough to be used at home on a daily basis, does not require a prescription and is cost-effective.

Safety

Structured Silver is remarkably safe. It can be used internally or in any orifice of the body – eyes, ears, nose, mouth, rectum or vagina.

If taken internally, it selectively kills pathogenic bacteria while leaving healthy bacteria (probiotics) unharmed. The way this selection happens is similar to the way probiotics are able to survive within the harsh environment of the stomach and digestive tract. Probiotics have a double layer of fatty protection on their outer edge, whereas pathogenic bacteria do not. This fatty layer protects probiotics from stomach acid, allowing them to grow and contribute to digestion. In the same say, this lipid bi-layer protects probiotics from the water-based silver product's antibacterial action.

According to the Merck Manual of Diagnosis and Therapy (5), silver is not considered to be a heavy metal and it does not accumulate in the brain.(3) In fact, it is the only metal that is not considered to be a heavy metal because it does not produce heavy metal poisoning.(6)

According to the IRIS report, silver is non-toxic at 5000mg/kg of body weight and 90-99 percent of ingested silver leaves the body within 24 hours.(7)

Additionally, silver is already being used in hospitals, space shuttles, washing machines, water filters and many other settings for its ability to control unwanted microbes. Yet it is so safe and non-toxic that it would take a spill of over 12 million gallons of 10 ppm silver before the EPA would consider it a reportable spill.(8) In contrast, less than one millionth of that amount of spilled bleach requires an EPA report!

Ingesting Silver is Normal

For the internal use of silver, many people feel nervous about swallowing it until they realize that they already do it every day.

Silver is ingested in many foods. Mushrooms contain silver concentrations as high as several hundred parts per billion. Most meats contain silver. According to World Health Organization estimates, people typically consume between 20 and 50 micrograms of silver on a daily basis.

Not surprisingly, silver is found in our bodily tissues. One of the highest concentrations of silver is within the platelets of our blood. This is interesting, as platelets are an essential part of the body's natural healing response.

Silver is also found in our drinking water, lakes and rivers. The EPA suggests that drinking water should contain less than 0.10 milligrams per liter of water (9) which translates roughly into 0.1 ppm. Note that this is for daily drinking water, which is measured in liters, whereas a 10 ppm silver supplement is taken only teaspoons at a time. The silver within Structured Silver is prepared for optimal benefit and does not require a high concentration.

Although we encounter silver on a daily basis through our diets and environment, not all forms of silver are the same. Some forms of silver can be poisonous, such as silver proteins, silver salts and industrial byproducts containing silver. It is important to distinguish products containing silver from one another. Always ask yourself, "Which form of silver is it?"

Preventative

As a result of its safety, Structured Silver can be used as a full-time preventive antimicrobial. It is excreted so quickly and thoroughly that regular small ingestions (two teaspoons twice daily) are typically recommended for general usage.

Unlike conventional antibiotics, which are only available by prescription and are typically not recommended for long-term use, Structured Silver is able to combat pathogens without creating resistance. This can be helpful for general use, for protection when traveling or for preventive use when visiting places with an elevated risk of infection.

For topical applications such as facial cleansing, hand disinfection or vaginal cleansing daily use is also safe.

Structured Silver Passes From the Body Unmetabolized

Not many substances pass through the body unmetabolized (a scientist's way of saying "it doesn't change between swallowing and excretion"), but Structured Silver does just that. This is an unusual characteristic for an antimicrobial. Pharmaceutical products that work by chemical action are typically consumed while killing germs within the body, one molecule at a time until the dose is fully utilized. In contrast, Structured Silver liquid's ability to work by physics without chemical consumption is a distinguishing characteristic that is surprising to those of the biochemistry paradigm.

The result is that Structured Silver is just as effective at disinfecting when it is leaving the body (killing the germs that cause bladder infections and urinary tract infections) as it was when it was swished in the mouth several hours earlier (killing the germs that cause gum disease, bad breath, cold sores, etc.) In between drinking and excretion, it will have been equally effective while circulating through the bloodstream (killing pathogens wherever the blood flows) or traveling through the digestive tract (killing pathogens like E. coli or Salmonella a person may have swallowed at lunchtime.)

For women who experience frequent bladder and urinary tract infections, this is welcome news. As urine gathers in the bladder and is excreted, the same silver that eliminated germs throughout the body will disinfect these organs as well.

Over 10 million bottles of newer silvers have been consumed in the last decade with not one confirmed adverse reaction. Additionally, uncountable amounts of the purer colloidal silvers have been safely consumed over the last one hundred years. This is largely connected to the fact that silver in the right form (pure, metallic and low concentration) passes through the body.

Topical Use

While Structured Silver is effective for internal cleansing, it is equally effective on the surface of the body. For example, pathogens can flourish on the skin within wrinkles, scrapes, pores, bites, cuticles, piercings and even burns such as sunburn. Prevention of small external infections can have a rapid effect. Structured Silver can be applied topically as a gel and as a liquid using a mister, gauze or soaking the skin.

Structured Silver makes a perfect skin conditioner because it does not contain alcohol or petroleum products. Alcohol can dry the skin, which can cause cracking and bleeding when used consistently. Petroleum based sanitizers can leave a greasy residue, causing a tacky feeling or flakes once the product has dried.

Skin can be damaged by many things, including wind, sun, makeup and detergent. The protective barrier that usually keeps our skin healthy comes from oils that are secreted by the skin, but as we get older we secrete less and less of these protective oils. By using Structured Silver gel on the skin one to four times a day, the skin will stay moist and a protective antibacterial barrier will be created to prevent disease from entering the skin.

The gel can also be combined with other routines and products on a daily basis. For example, it can be mixed with aloe vera at a 1:1 ratio and applied one to four times per day. For additional skin supplementation, amino acids, vitamin E or flax oil supplements can be helpful.

From Theory to Application

While background information about silver may be interesting, the real magic occurs when you first experience silver working in your own life. Thus, the remainder of this booklet has practical information for applying silver in the most common situations women encounter. After speaking with thousands of women before and after they began to use silver, I sincerely hope that this transcription of experience will also be of service to you.

While detail for specific situations is helpful, it is also helpful to start with a general recommendation for silver use. A rule of thumb, if you will. In most cases, a good plan is to drink two teaspoons of liquid silver twice per day (12 hours apart) and to apply gel or liquid topically as needed. There are more specific recommendations that are more helpful, but generally speaking, a good rule of thumb is: "two teaspoons twice per day; gel as needed."

For severe, life-threatening infections, doctors have recommended two ounces every six hours until there is evidence that the infection has been overcome.

Many people like to use gel for topical applications, but the liquid can be applied topically as well. Purse-sized spray containers, cotton balls, gauze and soaking are all easy ways to gain a topical benefit of silver using the liquid if a gel is unavailable. Both liquid and gel are great options for topical use.

For vaginal infections, a general recommendation is also helpful. I suggest consulting the following pages for greater detail, but here are some quick notes regarding vaginal use:

- To quickly control a vaginal infection, silver can be used as a douche. Two ounces of the product can be pumped intravaginally, held for 12 minutes and then released. Gel can then be applied to the surface.
- Structured Silver can help prevent vaginal infections. By putting gel on a tampon before inserting, you will receive antibacterial, antiviral, anti-mold and even anti-parasitic benefits. This method can be used for 30 minutes at a time, four hours apart.
- Liquid or gel can be used in a panty liner for an added layer of protection.
- In addition to keeping yeast and bacterial infections under control, when used as a personal lubricant on the surface of condoms, silver can kill viruses and sexually transmitted diseases.
- Silver can be used in the bathtub. Pour in four ounces and enjoy a warm bath for 25 minutes. This will cleanse the vagina and anus.

PART 2:
WOMEN'S ISSUES

The following list of female health concerns is presented in alphabetical order.

Bacterial infection of the vagina (Vaginosis)

Description: A bacteria-caused infection of the vagina and vulva.

Symptoms: Redness, itching, inflammation, bumps, irritation and burning when urinating. Usually causes a discharge with fishlike odor and is associated with itching and irritation.

Causes: Streptococcus, Garnerella, sexually transmitted diseases, lack of estrogen, poor hygiene and contamination from the rectum.

Recommendations:
- Structured Silver liquid: Drink a minimum of two teaspoons twice a day for prevention and treatment.
- Structured Silver gel: Apply to affected area two to five times a day for as long as needed.
- Structured Silver gel: Apply to a tampon and insert into the vagina for 90 minutes a day where the gel can stay in contact with the germs.
- Structured Silver douche: Use three ounces of Structured Silver liquid and mix it with three ounces of distilled water. Pump the solution into the vaginal cavity and hold for ten minutes, then release. This should be done once a day, for five days, or until symptoms are gone.
- Take daily probiotics (at least 8 billion active cultures) every day.
- Reduce dietary sugars and carbohydrates.
- Take large doses of antioxidants. This will help neutralize and clear the free radicals produced by the pathogens.

What you can expect: Numerous scientific studies show that silver can destroy the bacteria that cause vaginosis in under six minutes of contact. This means you can expect the liquid and gel to destroy the cause of vaginosis, as long as the silver stays in contact with the pathogen for six minutes. Most women feel noticeably better in one day and may return to normal in as little as two to five days.

Chlamydia (see also "Contamination from Sex")

Description: Chlamydia is a type of bacteria that is transferred by sexual contact. It destroys the tissues inside the vagina and returns when the immune system is depressed. It is also called "the clap."

Symptoms: Pain, inflammation, rash and tissue damage.

Cause: Bacteria inside vagina and surrounding area.

Recommendations:
- Structured Silver liquid: Drink two teaspoons twice a day for prevention.
- Structured Silver gel: Use as a personal lubricant on the male and female genitals prior to sex. It is a water-soluble gel that lubricates just like K-Y Jelly. Structured Silver gel will destroy the sexually transmitted diseases like gonorrhea, syphilis, HIV, herpes simplex and chlamydia.
- Use Structured Silver gel on the condom to lubricate and destroy the bacteria, viruses and yeast that may be transferred during intercourse.

Cramps

Description: Muscle cramps in vaginal wall and uterus.

Symptoms: Muscle cramps that result in pain and suffering.

Causes: Lack of oxygen in the muscles, muscle spasms, nerve irritation and toxins in the blood stream and muscles.

Recommendations:
- Structured Silver liquid: Drink two tablespoons twice a day to help destroy the toxins in the bloodstream.
- Structured Silver gel: Apply to the sore muscles twice daily.
- Take calcium and magnesium supplements.

Contamination from Sex

Description: Exchanging germs during sexual intercourse.

Symptoms: Infections of the genitalia and surrounding area from bacteria, viruses and yeast resulting tissue damage, itching, burning and long-term chronic disease.

Cause: Bacteria, viruses and yeast infecting the genitalia.

Recommendations:
- Structured Silver liquid: Drink two teaspoons twice a day for prevention.
- Structured Silver gel: Use as a personal lubricant on the male and female genitals prior to sex. It is a water-soluble gel that lubricates just like K-Y Jelly. Structured Silver gel will destroy the sexually transmitted diseases like gonorrhea, syphilis, HIV, herpes simplex and chlamydia.
- Use the gel on the condom to lubricate and destroy the bacteria, viruses and yeast that may be transferred during intercourse.

Endometriosis (see also "Painful Menstruation")

Description: Severe uterine pain during menstruation.

Symptoms: The main symptom of endometriosis is pain concentrated in the lower abdomen and may localize to one side of the abdomen or radiate pain to the thighs and low back. Other symptoms include sharp, throbbing, dull, nauseating, burning or shooting pains during dysmenorrheal (painful menstruation.) Endometriosis may be present for long or short term and may precede menstruation by several days or may accompany it. It usually subsides as menstruation tapers off. This severe pain may coexist with excessively heavy blood loss. On rare occasions nausea, vomiting, diarrhea, headache, dizziness or disorientation may occur.

Causes: Prostaglandins are inflammatory compounds that are released during menstruation and they cause the muscles of the uterus to contract. Sometimes, the uterus muscles constrict so much that the blood supply is compressed reducing the delivery of blood to the sensitive tissues of the endometrium. The absence of blood flow to the endometrium causes pain and cramping as the tissues die from the lack of blood. The uterus begins to contract in such a strong manner that the dead tissues are squeezed out of the uterus and out through the cervix and vagina. This temporary oxygen deprivation in the uterus is responsible for the cramps and pain. Silver makes dramatic improvements in wound healing and pain management inside the uterus. It also reduces inflammation, which can help reduce the cause of this painful disease.

Recommendations:
- Structured Silver liquid: Take a minimum of two teaspoons minimum twice a day for prevention and treatment.
- Structured Silver gel: Apply topically to affected area two to five times a day for as long as needed.
- Structured Silver gel: Apply to a tampon and insert into the vagina for 90 minutes a day where the gel can stay in contact with the germs.
- Structured Silver douche: Use three ounces of Structured Silver liquid and mix it with three ounces of distilled water. Pump the solution into the vaginal cavity and hold for ten

minutes, then release. This should be done once a day, for five days, or until symptoms are gone.
- Optional uses: Pour four ounces of liquid silver into a warm full tub of water, then bathe, soak and relax, flushing the silver water into the vaginal cavity. Twenty-five minutes is average for a muscle relaxing vaginal flush in the tub.

Additional Products: Herbal products that help reduce inflammation and pain and improve hormone balance include black cohosh, blue vervain, Suma and white willow.

Gonorrhea (see Contamination from Sex)

Recommendations:
- Structured Silver liquid: Drink two teaspoons twice a day for prevention.
- Structured Silver gel: Use as a personal lubricant on the male and female genitals prior to sex. It is a water-soluble gel that lubricates just like K-Y Jelly. Structured Silver gel will destroy the sexually transmitted diseases like gonorrhea, syphilis, HIV, herpes simplex and chlamydia.
- Use the gel on the condom to lubricate and destroy the bacteria, viruses and yeast that may be transferred during intercourse.

Herpes Virus (see also "Viral Vaginal Infections")

Description: Herpes virus infections within and outside the vagina.

Symptoms: Water blisters inside and outside the vagina producing extremely painful conditions depending on the severity of the lesions of blisters.

Causes: Herpes virus.

Recommendations:

- Structured Silver liquid: swallow two teaspoons at minimum twice a day for prevention and treatment.
- Structured Silver gel: Apply topically to affected area two to five times a day for as long as needed.
- Structured Silver gel: Apply to the finger or swab and inserted into the vagina for 90 minutes a day where the gel can stay in contact with the germs.
- Structured Silver douche: Use three ounces of Structured Silver liquid and mix it with three ounces of distilled water. Pump the solution into the vaginal cavity and hold for ten minutes, then release. This should be done once a day, for five days, or until symptoms are gone.
- Take daily probiotics (at least 8 billion active cultures) every day.
- Reduce dietary sugars and carbohydrates.
- By taking large doses of antioxidants you can expect to neutralize and clear the free radicals produced by the pathogens.

What you can expect: Silver can destroy the virus that causes infections in under six minutes. This means you can expect the liquid and gel to destroy the cause of viral infections as long as the silver stays in contact with the pathogen for six minutes. Most women feel noticeably better in one day and may return to normal in as little as two to five days.

Herpes Simplex (Fever Blisters)

Recommendations:
- Structured Silver liquid: Take a minimum of two teaspoons at minimum twice a day for prevention and treatment.
- Structured Silver gel: Apply topically to affected area two to five times a day for as long as needed.
- The sooner the gel gets on the blister the faster it will heal. If you get the gel on the wound (and keep it moist with gel) in the first four hours that the blister erupts it will stop it from erupting and shrink back to normal without rupturing

or spreading. The key is to get silver gel on the wound as soon as you feel a pinch or sting and keep the gel on every 30 minutes for the first four hours.

Hysterectomy, Pelvic Inflammatory Disease

Description: Chronic inflammation of the pelvic region due to ongoing infections.

Symptoms: Long term inflammation and infections of the vagina, vulva, uterus and surrounding tissues. It may be painful for a short or long period of time and is aggravated by urination, sexual activity or yeast overgrowth.

Symptoms: Extreme pain, inflammation and possible nausea, with fever.

Causes: Bacteria, viruses and yeast.

Recommendations:
- Structured Silver liquid: Drink two teaspoons twice a day for prevention or drink two tablespoons twice a day for severe conditions.
- Structured Silver gel: Apply to the affected and painful area at least twice a day to destroy the pathogens that cause the pain and infection.
- Silver douche: Use three ounces of Structured Silver liquid and mix it with three ounces of distilled water and pump the solution into the vaginal cavity and hold for ten minutes, then release. This should be done once a day, for five days, or until symptoms are gone.
- Optional uses: Pour four ounces of liquid silver into a warm full tub of water, then bathe, soak and relax, flushing the silver water into the vaginal cavity. Twenty-five minutes is average for a muscle relaxing vaginal flush in the tub.

Human Papillomavirus (HPV) (see also "Viral Vaginal Infections")

Description: A viral infection, usually afflicting the cervix, which can damage cellular DNA and cause cancer of the cervix.

Symptoms: Most of the time there are no symptoms except lab tests performed by the doctor. There is no real treatment from a doctor until the tissue damage by the virus has become cancerous. At this point surgery is performed. Structured Silver liquid (douche) and gel on a tampon give the woman a method of destroying the cause of the abnormal cells and possibly preventing the cause of the cancer.

Cause: Human Papillomavirus (HPV)

Recommendations:
- Structured Silver liquid: Drink a minimum of two teaspoons twice a day for prevention and treatment.
- Structured Silver gel: Apply to the tip of a tampon and insert into the vagina for 90 minutes a day where the gel can stay in contact with the germs.
- Silver douche: Use three ounces of Structured Silver liquid and mix it with three ounces of distilled water. Pump the solution into the vaginal cavity and hold for ten minutes, then release. This should be done once a day, for five days, or until symptoms are gone.
- Take daily probiotics (at least 8 billion active cultures) every day.
- Reduce dietary sugars and carbohydrates.
- Take large doses of antioxidants. This will help neutralize and clear free radicals produced by the pathogens.

What you can expect: Silver can destroy the virus's ability to replicate, reducing the level of viral infection over time. Silver can inhibit both types of viral replication (RNA and DNA.) Most women feel noticeably better in one day and may return to normal in as little as two to five days.

Infertility

Description: Inability to get pregnant or carry a pregnancy to full term.

Causes: Approximately 10 percent of couples have difficulty conceiving and 25 percent of the time it is the male that is infertile. Genetic factors, diabetes reduces blood flow, pituitary, hypothalamus, pituitary problems reduce fertility. In addition, the following toxins have been shown to cause infertility: glues, volatile solvents, silicones, pesticides and chemical dusts. Tobacco smokers are 60 percent more likely to be infertile because smoking increases the chances of miscarriage by 30 percent. Infections of the blood, vagina, cervix, vulva or male organs can contribute to reproductive organ infections, which interfere with fertility. (Silver can reduce this problem by destroying bacteria, viruses and fungus that cause the infections, including sexually transmitted diseases.)

Recommendations:
- Structured Silver liquid: A minimum of two teaspoons twice a day.
- Structured Silver gel: Use during intercourse to prevent sexually transmitted diseases, yeast infections and bacterial vaginosis.
- Structured Silver gel: Apply to the vaginal opening and male genitals daily to reduce pathogens.
- Remember that silver will destroy the bacteria, viruses and yeast if it stays in contact with the germ for six to ten minutes.
- Follow your doctor's recommendations concerning ovulation, supplements, stimulants, hormones etc.

Menopause

Description: Hormone changes that produce physiologic, behavioral and mental changes.

Symptoms: Mental anxiety, delusion, hot flashes, pain, cessation of menstruation, ageing and skin degeneration.

Causes: Reduction in the female hormones resulting in changes in the normal physiologic functions, mental well being and behavioral adjustments to the changes in hormones. Some times bacteria or fungus can negatively affect the hormone balance from the ovaries. With the changes in hormone levels the skin loses some of its ability to maintain flexible, regenerative abilities.

Recommendations:
- Structured Silver liquid: Drink a minimum of two teaspoons twice a day to prevent and maintain wellness.
- Structured Silver gel: Apply to the face, head, neck and all other skin areas to help reduce bacterial, viral and fungal infections. The gel helps with existing wounds and long-term scars. Apply to these wounds or scars twice daily for three months and expect significant improvement in wound healing and reduction of existing scars, while preventing the cause of acne and premature aging.

Painful Menstruation, Dysmenorrhea, Menstrual Cramps, Endometriosis and PMS

Description: Severe uterine pain during menstruation.

Symptoms: The main symptom of dysmenorrheal (painful menstruation) is pain concentrated in the lower abdomen and may localize to one side of the abdomen or radiate pain to the thighs and lower back. Various types of pain – sharp, throbbing, dull, nauseating, burning or shooting – are noted during dysmenorrhea. Dysmenorrhea may precede menstruation by several days or may accompany it and usually subsides as menstruation tapers off. The severe pain may coexist with excessively heavy blood loss. On rare occasions nausea, vomiting, diarrhea, headache, dizziness or disorientation may occur.

Causes: Prostaglandins are inflammatory compounds that are released during menstruation. They cause the muscles of the uterus to constrict so much that blood supply is compressed, reducing the delivery of blood to the sensitive tissues of the endometrium. The absence of blood flow to the endometrium causes pain and cramping as the tissues die from the lack of blood. The uterus begins to contract in such a strong manner that the dead tissues are squeezed out of the uterus and out through the cervix and vagina. This temporary oxygen deprivation in the uterus is responsible for the cramps and pain. Silver makes dramatic improvements in wound healing and pain management inside the uterus. It also reduces inflammation, which can help reduce the cause of this painful menstruation.

Recommendations:
- Structured Silver liquid: Drink a minimum of two teaspoons twice a day for prevention and treatment.
- Structured Silver gel: Apply topically to affected area two to five times a day for as long as needed.
- Structured Silver gel: Apply to a tampon and inserted into the vagina for 90 minutes a day.
- Silver douche: Use three ounces of Structured Silver liquid and mix it with three ounces of distilled water. Pump the solution into the vaginal cavity and hold for ten minutes, then release. This should be done once a day, for five days, or until symptoms are gone.
- Optional uses: Pour four ounces of liquid silver into a warm full tub of water, then bathe, soak and relax, flushing the silver water into the vaginal cavity. Twenty-five minutes is average for a muscle relaxing vaginal flush in the tub.

Additional Products: Herbal products that help reduce inflammation and pain and improve hormone balance include black cohosh, blue vervain, Suma and white willow.

Premenstrual Syndrome (PMS) (see "Painful Menstruation")

Sexually Transmitted Diseases (see also "Contamination from Sex")

Recommendations:
- Structured Silver liquid: Drink two teaspoons at minimum twice a day for prevention.
- Use Structured Silver gel as a personal lubricant, on the male and female genitals prior to sex. It is a water-soluble gel that lubricates just like K-Y Jelly. Structured Silver gel will destroy the sexually transmitted diseases like gonorrhea, syphilis, HIV, herpes simplex and chlamydia.
- Use Structured Silver gel on the condom to lubricate and destroy the bacteria, viruses and yeast that may be transferred during intercourse.

Skin Infections, Acne and Mastitis

Description: Infections on and under the skin.

Symptoms: Infections under the skin causing the inflammation and the destruction of healthy skin tissues resulting in pustules, cysts, boils and inflamed painful tissues.

Causes: Bacteria, viruses and fungus that infects healthy skin topically and under the surface of the skin.

Recommendations:
- Structured Silver liquid: Drink two teaspoons at minimum twice a day for wellness.
- Structured Silver gel: Apply to infected areas at least twice a day (up to six times a day) to destroy the cause of the infection. Alternately, a small spray bottle, easily carried in a purse or backpack, can be used on the skin throughout the day.
- For the face: Apply Structured Silver gel as soon as you leave the shower and have pat-dried your face. Then wait

two minutes for the gel to penetrate the skin, after which you can apply makeup.
- For other skin infections like mastitis or athletes foot: Apply the gel to the skin twice a day or more as needed.
- If the gel can penetrate the skin and get the source of the infection, it will kill the bacteria in six minutes.

Syphilis (see also "Contamination from Sex")

Recommendations:
- Structured Silver liquid: Drink a minimum of two teaspoons twice a day for prevention.
- Use Structured Silver gel as a personal lubricant on the male and female genitals prior to sex. It is a water-soluble gel that lubricates just like K-Y Jelly. Structured Silver gel will destroy the sexually transmitted diseases like gonorrhea, syphilis, HIV, herpes simplex and chlamydia.
- Use Structured Silver gel on the condom to lubricate and destroy the bacteria, viruses and yeast that may be transferred during intercourse.

Urinary Tract Infection (UTI)

Description: A urinary infection (UTI) is bacterial infection that affects any part of the urinary tract. The kidney, ureters and bladder are adversely affected by invading bacteria that multiply in the urine.

Symptoms: The most common symptom is pain and burning during urination. Other symptoms are urinating for frequently and an abnormal urgency to urinate without vaginal discharge.

A kidney infection may occur with pain in the lower back or flank area, with possible more serious symptoms of chills, nausea, vomiting and high fever.

A bladder infection (called cystitis) is usually associated with abdominal pain, incontinence, blood in urine, pus in urine, inability to urinate despite the urge and malaise.

Causes: Bacteria, viruses and fungus that infect the genital area.

Recommendations:
- Structured Silver liquid: Drink two ounces every hour for four hours. Since silver destroys the bacteria that cause the infection in six minutes, it is important to absorb large amounts of silver for four hours. In this way the silver can wash through the kidneys and pool in the bladder. Silver passes through the body unchanged, meaning that the silver that pools in the bladder will still kill the bacteria in the kidneys, bladder and urethra.
- Structured Silver gel: Apply topically twice a day to affected area twice a day or as needed.
- Take 8 billion active cultures of probiotics that contain acidophilus and bifidus daily.
- Take large doses of antioxidants. This will help neutralize and clear free radicals produced by the pathogens.
- Cranberry is terrific at helping reduce bladder infections.

What you can expect: Silver can destroy the bacteria that cause infections in the urinary tract in under six minutes. This means you can expect the liquid and gel to destroy the cause of the UTI as long as the silver stays in contact with the pathogen for six minutes. Most women feel noticeably better in two hours and may return to normal in as little as four to six hours.

Vaginal Bleeding (see also "Painful Menstruation")

Recommendations:
- Structured Silver gel: Apply topically to affected area two to five times a day for as long as needed.

- Structured Silver gel: Apply to a tampon and inserted into the vagina for 90 minutes a day where the gel can stay in contact with the wounds in the vagina.
- Silver douche: Use three ounces of Structured Silver liquid and mix it with three ounces of distilled water. Pump the solution into the vaginal cavity and hold for ten minutes, then release. This should be done once a day, for five days, or until symptoms are gone.
- Structured Silver liquid: Take a minimum of two teaspoons twice a day for prevention and treatment.
- Optional uses: Pour four ounces of liquid silver into a warm full tub of water, then bathe, soak and relax, flushing the silver water into the vaginal cavity. Twenty-five minutes is average for a muscle relaxing vaginal flush in the tub.

Additional Products: Herbal products that help reduce inflammation and pain and improve hormone balance include black cohosh, blue vervain, Suma and white willow.

Vaginal Dryness

Recommendations:
- Structured Silver gel should be applied twice a day or as many times as needed to lubricate the vulva and vagina and to help prevent infections, inflammation and disease.
- Structured Silver gel can be applied to the penis, vulva and vagina or on the condom to help lubricate during intercourse. Apply liberally, knowing that it does not contain any alcohol (so it won't irritate the sensitive tissues of the vagina) and it does not contain any petroleum (so it will not cause stickiness, greasiness or macerate the vulva.)

Vaginal Infections, Trichomoniasis, Chlamydia, Viral Vaginitis/Vulvitis and Vulvodynia

Recommendations:
- Structured Silver liquid: Drink a minimum of two teaspoons twice a day for prevention.
- Use Structured Silver gel as a personal lubricant on the male and female genitals prior to sex. It is a water-soluble gel that lubricates just like K-Y Jelly. Structured Silver gel will destroy the sexually transmitted diseases like gonorrhea, syphilis, HIV, herpes simplex and chlamydia.
- Use Structured Silver gel on the condom to lubricate and destroy the bacteria, viruses and yeast that may be transferred during intercourse.

Vaginitis

Description: Inflammation and irritation of the vagina caused by yeast or bacteria causing pain, itching and discomfort in the vaginal area.

Symptoms: Can produce redness, inflammation, itching, burning, discomfort when urinating, possibly a foul vaginal odor and may be associated with abnormal discharge or pain during intercourse.

Additional notes:
- Candida causes watery, white cottage cheese like vaginal discharge, which is irritating to the vagina and the surrounding skin.
- Bacterial causes are usually associated with a fishlike odor and is associated with itching and irritation, but not during intercourse.
- Viruses can cause profuse discharge with a strong fishlike odor, pain upon urination, painful intercourse and inflammation of the external genitals.

Causes: Candida (yeast), Gardnerella (bacteria), Streptococcus (bacteria), Herpes (virus), Trichomonas (parasite).

Recommendations:
- Structured Silver liquid: Drink at minimum two teaspoons twice a day for one week or until symptoms subside.
- Structured Silver gel: Apply topically twice a day to affected area. You can also apply Structured Silver gel to the tip of a tampon and insert into the vagina for 90 minutes a day for a week.
- Silver douche: Use three ounces of Structured Silver liquid and mix it with three ounces of distilled water. Pump the solution into the vaginal cavity and hold for ten minutes, then release. This should be done once per day for five days or until symptoms are gone.
- Stop eating sugars, yeasts and breads that feed the yeast.
- Take 8 billion active cultures of probiotics that contain acidophilus and bifidus daily.
- Take large doses of antioxidants. This will help neutralize and clear free radicals produced by the pathogens.

What you can expect: Structured Silver can destroy bacteria, viruses, trichomonas and yeast in under ten minutes. This means you can expect the liquid and gel to destroy the cause of vaginitis as long as the Structured Silver stays in contact with the pathogen for ten minutes. The parasite trichomonas may take six weeks to eliminate. Most women feel noticeably better in one day and may return to normal in as little as two to five days.

Viral Vaginal Infections

Description: Viruses (like herpes) that reside in the vaginal cavity and surrounding skin, cervix and uterus.

Symptoms: About one week after infection, water blisters appear on the genital region and are associated with tenderness, swollen glands and fever. The water blisters are extremely painful and heal in about three weeks unless silver is used. With silver, wound healing is as much as three times faster (one week).

Causes: Viruses (herpes)

Recommendations:
- Structured Silver liquid: Swallow two teaspoons at minimum twice a day for prevention and treatment.
- Structured Silver gel: Apply topically to affected area two to five times a day for as long as needed.
- Structured Silver gel: Apply to a finger or swab and insert into the vagina where the gel can stay in contact with the germs.
- Silver douche: Use three ounces of Structured Silver liquid and mix it with three ounces of distilled water. Pump the solution into the vaginal cavity and hold for ten minutes, then release. This should be done once a day, for five days, or until symptoms are gone.
- Take daily probiotics (at least 8 billion active cultures) every day.
- Reduce dietary sugars and carbohydrates.
- Take large doses of antioxidants. This will help neutralize and clear free radicals produced by the pathogens.

What you can expect: Silver can inhibit the replication of viruses, resulting in a gradual reduction in the viral load. Most women feel noticeably better in one day and may return to normal in as little as two to five days.

Yeast Infections (Candida)

Description: Yeast that has infected the vagina, cervix, uterus or vulvar opening resulting in tissue damage on the affected areas.

Symptoms: Redness, irritation, flaking skin, foul odor, itching, burning, and/or discomfort when urinating or during intercourse. May be associated with abnormal discharge. Usually causes a watery, white, cottage cheese like vaginal discharge, which is irritating to the vagina and surrounding skin.

Causes: Yeast (Candida)

Recommendations:
- Structured Silver liquid: Drink a minimum of two teaspoons twice a day for one week or until symptoms subside.
- Structured Silver gel: Apply topically twice a day to affected area. Apply Structured Silver gel to the tip of a tampon and insert into the vagina for 90 minutes a day for a week.
- Silver douche: Use three ounces of Structured Silver liquid and mix it with three ounces of distilled water. Pump the solution into the vaginal cavity and hold for ten minutes, then release. This should be done once a day, for five days, or until symptoms are gone.
- Stop eating sugars, yeasts and breads that feed the yeast.
- Take 8 billion active cultures of probiotics that contain acidophilus and bifidus daily.
- Take large doses of antioxidants. This will help neutralize and clear free radicals produced by the pathogens.
- Caprylic acid has been shown to help reduce intestinal yeast and may help if the yeast is systemic.

What you can expect: Silver can destroy yeast in under ten minutes. This means you can expect the liquid and gel to destroy the cause of yeast infections as long as the silver stays in contact with the pathogen for ten minutes. Most women feel noticeably better in one day and may return to normal in as little as two to five days.

Wellness

Description: The habits that promote constant wellness and disease-free living, which promotes a wholeness and foundation for happy living.

Symptoms: Healthy body systems, normal constant wellness, balanced and self-reliant immunity and the ability to defend against environmental pathogens.

Causes: The causes of wellness are numerous: a positive attitude, healthy genetics, eating correctly, sleeping sufficiently to recharge, exercise, regular cleansing, reduction of stress and supplementing where there are deficiencies or greater needs. Silver is the perfect supplement for healthy living because it destroys the cause of most disease-causing bacteria, viruses and yeast. By taking silver daily it reduces the workload on an already overworked immune system. Silver can be your first line of defense because it supports a healthy immune system and works directly on any part of the body that is infected, weakened or in need of healing. By taking silver two teaspoons twice a day you are promoting wellness. In the event you need to use more, it is safe to double or quadruple the amount for a month. The gel is magnificent because it works wherever you apply it, inside or outside the body.

Recommendations:
- Structured Silver liquid: Drink two teaspoons twice a day for prevention and double it when there is more demand.
- Structured Silver gel: Apply to wounds, scratches, scrapes, vaginal infections, the mouth, nose, throat or wherever there is need to destroy germs. The gel can be safely used as many as one to ten times a day for three months at a time, then return to normal or near normal usage.

PART 3:
ADDITIONAL HEALTH ISSUES

This list of health issues is not exclusive to women, though women often ask about them more frequently than men.

Aging

There are many reasons why we may age prematurely – a liver that doesn't function properly, tissues that degenerate too quickly, a sedentary lifestyle, a lack of nutrients and the toxins all around us.

Yeast is one of the main components in premature aging. We have yeast between our toes and in our intestines. It's found anywhere there is a warm, moist area and destroys one cell at a time. Likewise, bacteria can cause tissue damage. Silver prevents premature aging by killing bacteria, viruses and yeast.

Drink one teaspoon of Structured Silver liquid twice a day for wellness and prevention. If you are sick, drink two teaspoons or more twice a day. Structured Silver gel can also be applied to specific areas topically one to three times a day. Additional benefits can come from using freeform amino acids, vitamins, minerals and essential fatty acids.

Appetite Suppressant

Many people who suffer from overeating say they just can't seem to satisfy their appetite. Food craving can be increased by an intestinal yeast growth that puts neurotoxins into the blood stream. This creates damage everywhere the blood circulates, including the brain. Yeast is fed by sugar and causes the body to crave more sugar.

Structured Silver liquid will not directly control your appetite nor suppress it. However, if you have a yeast infection, Structured Silver can kill the yeast in your intestines, decreasing neurotoxins and food craving.

Structured Silver should be considered for any dietary plan. One teaspoon twice a day will help maintain wellness. A digestive cleanse will also be beneficial.

Chronic Fatigue Syndrome

Chronic fatigue syndrome has a number of different causes – viral, bacterial, hormonal or parasitic. Important identifying factors include muscle and joint aches, stiffness and fatigue. It can also affect hearing and eyesight.

Two tablespoons of Structured Silver can be taken two or three times a day for relief. Gel can be applied or sprayed on sore muscles once or twice a day as needed for aches and pains. Structured Silver liquid drops can be used in the eyes and ears as well.

Many people suffering from Epstein bar virus or mononucleosis have taken Structured Silver to help restore their energy. Additional products to help with chronic fatigue are coenzyme Q10 and freeform amino acids.

Cuticles

For cuticle care, soak your fingers in Structured Silver liquid for 30 minutes or apply Structured Silver directly. For cracked, dry cuticles, cover the hands with rubber gloves after applying the silver to seal in moisture.

Depression

Depression can occur for a lot of different reasons, including biochemical and hormonal imbalances. A sedentary lifestyle can also lead to depression.

When a person has a depressed system, their chemistry needs to get back into balance. This isn't always easy. It requires a healthy diet and exercise. It has been found that people exercising 90 minutes a week over the course of eight weeks were able to control depression better than by taking antidepressant pharmaceutical drugs.

Bacterial and viral infections can have an effect on depression as well. Drinking one teaspoon of Structured Silver twice daily can keep these infections under control. St. John's Wort can help with mild to moderate depression and coenzyme Q10 can help with energy. A digestive parasite cleanse combined with Structured Silver can also improve depression by taking some of the toxins out of the intestinal system. Structured Silver liquid can be taken one to two teaspoons one to three times a day.

Eyes

There are many problems that can develop within the eyes, both bacterial and viral. Most of them come from the outside, except for a few circulatory problems.

Spray or drop two or three drops of silver liquid directly into the eyes one to four times a day and drink two teaspoons twice a day for one week, or until the problem is remedied. On a long-term basis, one teaspoon twice a day will suffice.

If you kill the bacteria and viruses on the surface of the eye you will reduce redness, inflammation and itchiness. Hopefully proper tearing will be restored and you will have an eye that has a chance to heal itself fully.

After using Structured Silver, you should expect visible and noticeable difference in the first hour, with substantial improvements within two hours. Lutein, blueberry and antioxidants also help.

Facial Mask

Most facial masks only peel the dead skin cells off the surface of the face. Structured Silver can actually remove the toxins.

I recommend a powdered clay mix with added Structured Silver. When the clay is applied to the skin in liquid form, the silver will remove the bacteria while firming and tightening the skin. The clay will remove oils and detoxify the skin, destroying the causes of acne and blemishes. Supplement by drinking one teaspoon of Structured Silver liquid twice a day.

Facial Peel

Some people use a facial peel to get down to the new and youthful layers of skin. These peels use harsh chemicals, basically burning the skin at the very top layer of its cells. By applying Structured Silver gel after a facial peel you'll experience quick improvements, better color and reduced pain and damage. You'll also get longer results with better cellular structure. One teaspoon of liquid Structured Silver should also be taken daily.

Facial Treatment

Structured Silver can be used as a facial treatment to help with regeneration of damaged cells and wound management. It can also treat acne, infections, blemishes and premature aging. Large groups of women have co-op purchased cases of silver with fantastic cosmetic results.

You will get the deepest Structured Silver penetration by washing the face with a mild soap, patting it dry and then applying the gel or spraying the liquid to the skin while it is still moist. The gel or liquid can also be applied after steaming the face. This will open up the sweat glands and hair follicles, allowing the Structured Silver to get deeper into the skin. This allows Structured Silver particles to prevent infections and improve wound healing at the same time. It will also help prevent premature aging at the cellular level. You should also drink a minimum of one teaspoon of liquid Structured Silver twice a day.

If you have sensitive skin, you will find Structured Silver liquid and gel reduce inflammation, swelling, puffiness and allergies.

Hand Disinfection and Restoration

As we age, our hands are exposed to sunlight, cleansing agents and drying agents. The skin gets wrinkled and damaged. By drinking one teaspoon of liquid Structured Silver twice a day, the silver will enter the red blood cells and work from the inside out of the capillary system. Applying Structured Silver gel one to four times a day will benefit the topical layers of the skin.

The same application of silver replaces the role of alcohol or petroleum based hand sanitizers. Alcohol based products dry out the skin and can cause cracking of the skin. Petroleum based products leave a greasy feeling or flaking as the product dries. In contrast, the silver gel can comfortably sanitize hands for four hours without staining or other undesirable effects.

Itching

Itching and scaling can occur for many reasons, including bacteria, viruses, funguses and allergies. Regardless of the cause, dry skin is always a factor. Structured Silver gel or liquid will reduce pain, inflammation, itching and scaling. Additionally, it may remove the cause of itching. The gel or liquid can be applied to children and adults of any age.

Itching in the crotch is a common source of discomfort. If you live in a warm, humid or tropical climate, you may have a fungal or bacterial infection that grows in the warm, moist folds of the skin, including the groin. Simple application of the Structured Silver gel or liquid twice daily should keep it under control. For more aggressive cases, it can be used five times a day. In addition, at least one teaspoon of Structured Silver liquid should also be taken orally twice a day.

Lips

Many people suffer from chapped lips, the herpes virus (cold sores) or the lead in their lipstick. Placing Structured Silver gel on the lips every night will help to improve the lips and help to prevent damage. In addition, drink a minimum of one teaspoon of Structured Silver liquid twice a day. Cold sores respond quickly and no blister will occur if, at very first sign of cold sore, the liquid is in constant contact for 30 minutes. A gauze or swab can be helpful for maintaining constant contact.

If you use lip balm, it is easy to create your own silver lip balm. By adding a little bit of heat, you can melt your preferred lip balm. Add a small amount of liquid silver and then let the balm re-thicken. This will allow you to enjoy the benefits of silver each time you moisten your lips.

Makeup Irritation

When people put on makeup every day it often begins to irritate their skin. The skin may become red and itchy. Rashes can form. To neutralize this problem, apply Structured Silver gel and drink one teaspoon of Structured Silver liquid on a daily basis.

In addition, when the makeup is removed, soak a cotton ball with silver and wipe the face clean. This will neutralize pathogens that may aggravate or irritate the skin. It will also help with pain, redness and skin regeneration.

To add another layer of protection, Structured Silver should be applied at night before bed. Hypoallergenic makeup will also prevent irritation problems.

Structured Silver can be used in addition to, or in place of, makeup base. After you wash your face, apply a think layer of Structured Silver gel. Wait two minutes for it to dry and then apply your base. This will give you protection against acne, blemishes and infections from mold, bacteria and viruses.

Some women use the Structured Silver gel as their base and natural coloring. This approach can replace damaging makeup and allergenic topical cleansing, as it washes clean with water.

MRSA, Staph

On any given day in America there are 30,000 new cases of MRSA. This is a bacterial staphylococcus infection that has become resistant to our antibiotics. It can affect the skin, eyes or any other part of the body. It can be fatal.

Structured Silver has been tested and documented to destroy MRSA and staph infections. To prevent these infections, drink one tablespoon of Structured Silver liquid twice a day and apply the gel to the hands at least twice a day. MRSA infections are serious so treat with up to two ounces every six hours in addition to any conventional antibiotics prescribed by medical industry.

MRSA can enter any wound and all of us have some form of staph bacteria on our skin at any given time. By using public restrooms, shaking hands, hugging, kissing or any other skin-to-skin contact, you may be at risk of getting or sharing staph MRSA infections.

Nails

When Structured Silver comes in contact with nail fungus (fingers or toes), it will kill it within minutes. The problem is getting underneath the nail. If possible, get through the nail and clear out as much fungus as possible with a blunt instrument. The nail fungus can then be treated by soaking the toe or finger in Structured Silver liquid for 30 minutes every other day. A finger cot can be filled half full with silver gel and stretched over the infected toe or finger. This will push the silver into the fungus. Do this for 30 minutes every other day, until the infection is gone.

If you can't get the silver through the nail, file down the top layer of the nail until it becomes water-soluble. This will allow the silver to reach the fungus and kill it. It will take several months for the nail to grow out completely.

Neck Firming

When a person ages, the skin can stretch due to the loss of elastin and collagen. By applying Structured Silver topically to the neck, you will remove the fungus and bacteria that may reside in the dead skin cells or wrinkles of the neck. The wrinkles will stop growing deeper and you will have a more youthful-looking skin. In this way, you'll have better skin texture. To achieve these benefits, put Structured Silver gel in the refrigerator, take it out and apply while cold one to four times a day.

Personal Lubricant

Personal lubricant can be used to lubricate joints of the elbow, armpits or anywhere skin is rubbing together and causing a rash. It is most commonly used, however, on condoms or for vaginal dryness. By using Structured Silver gel as a personal lubricant during sex, you will also destroy bacteria, viruses and mold – protecting both you and your sexual partner from sexually transmitted infections. It will also reduce the inflammation, swelling and pain associated with skin rubbing against skin.

Rosacea

Rosacea is a form of bacteria that grows on the nose, making it red and swollen with pimples. This can leave very large scars. Because it is difficult to treat, doctors generally prescribe antibiotics.

Rather than using antibiotics, you can drink two teaspoons of Structured Silver liquid twice a day and apply the gel or spray the liquid four times daily. Wash the nose lightly between each application. You should see a reduction of redness within the first two hours and a reduction of pimples in the first day.

Scars

A scar is formed when the skin is damaged and the immune system pulls it back together. The scar is made up of a thickened layer of skin. Scarring can be minimized by drinking at least one teaspoon of Structured Silver liquid twice a day and applying Structured Silver gel directly to the wound two to four times a day. The silver will keep the wound moist and remove bacteria, mold and viruses, which helps the healing process.

Structured Silver gel can also be applied directly to scars and stretch marks, softening the skin and reducing scar size. For severe, highly inflamed or keloid scars, apply the gel and cover it with plastic wrap or a sterile gauze bandage.

If you have open wounds, you should apply gel more regularly. If the wound is a MRSA infection, apply Structured Silver gel every two hours to keep it moist.

Travel Kit

Everybody needs a little help when they're traveling. When you're away from home, you'll want to take Structured Silver with you. There are a lot of reasons for this. Aside from being dehydrated or possibly being far from a hospital (or, at least, an affordable one), contact with unusual pathogens is typically higher while traveling.

For example, you can get salmonella from any type of food, from shaking hands and touching your eye, from licking your finger at a restaurant, from using a public toilet or from turning a door knob in a public building. These are some of the reasons that you'll want Structured Silver.

The point is very simple: take Structured Silver on your trips. Take at least two teaspoons of the liquid twice daily, apply the gel twice a day to your hands and while the gel is still wet on your hands, rub a little on the inside of your nostrils to help protect while you inhale. From experience, it is best to take more than you feel you will personally need – the people you travel with or meet may NEED your extra supply!

If you're traveling on a cruise ship, when you get on board you'll find that they almost always have hand sanitizer. If you use their hand sanitizer, in two days you're likely to have alcohol-burned hands. They will be cracked, dried, possibly bleeding and ready for infection. Instead, try Structured Silver gel. Another reason to take Structured Silver is that boats are filled with mold. No matter how well they are cleaned, ships are wet and mold grows. If you take Structured Silver with you and spray a little in your nose each day and put it on your hands, you'll go a long way towards preventing the mold from causing health problems.

Frequently Asked Questions Some Simple Answers to Common Questions

These questions have been asked thousands of times by newcomers to Structured Silver. For your convenience, here are simple answers:

Q: Why have liquid and gel?
A: The liquid can be used in all internal and topical applications. Some people prefer the gel for topical application. The gel is made of water, silver and a gelling agent, whereas the liquid is made of only water and silver.

Q: What's up with the ppm (parts per million)?
A: What is essential to note is that "more ppm" does not equate to "stronger or better silver." If Structured Silver worked by chemical action or molecular math alone, like a silver colloid product, higher concentrations would be important. But since Structured Silver works on pathogens through several mechanisms of action, "more silver" does not equal "works better."

Restated, higher concentrations do not necessarily kill more germs. If this wasn't true, we could just swallow silver coins and be done with it.

As an aside, the cost of silver as a raw material in Structured Silver is such a small fraction that it doesn't affect the choice of ppm at all. 10 ppm is chosen as the liquid's concentration because of its broad-spectrum efficacy.

Q: What is the shelf life?
A: Officially, two years. Given that it is a stable solution, it may be good for much longer than that.

Q: Does it need to be refrigerated?
A: No, room temperature is fine.

Q: Where is it made?
A: It is made in the United States under strict levels of quality control and manufacturing standards.

Q: Who can take Structured Silver?
A: Anyone can take silver, but the children under 75 pounds should take half the adult doses. Children under age one should take one-third the normal dose. By the way, the normal adult dose of the Structured Silver liquid is two teaspoons twice a day.

Q: When is the best time to take Structured Silver?
A: Take it at a time where you will not forget to take it. The best time to take it for daily prevention is two teaspoons twice a day, morning and night.

Q: Does Structured Silver affect my other medications, food, beverages, etc.?
A: No, it can be taken with anything except salt. The chloride ion binds with the silver and can neutralize some of the silver.

Q: Are there any contraindications using Structured Silver with any prescription products?
A: Don't mix Structured Silver with salt. The chloride ion binds with the silver and removes the silver's benefits. Other than that, there are no contraindications. If you are concerned about this, take the Structured Silver one hour before or after you take other medications or foods, holding the liquid in your mouth for five minutes before swallowing.

Q: Is it better to take Structured Silver with food or on an empty stomach?
A: If you take silver on an empty stomach there will be less salt to interfere with it. If you take it on an empty stomach you will

also absorb the silver about 15 minutes faster than if you take it with food.

Q: Should Structured Silver be used daily or just when I have a problem?
A: Structured Silver is designed to be used daily as a preventative. Two teaspoons of the liquid form taken twice a day is the normal dose. In gel form, it should be used twice a day or as needed. When a person has a more dramatic need they can double this dose and in some severe cases people have successfully taken four ounces per day for up to two weeks.

Q: How does Structured Silver support immune function?
A: Structured Silver benefits the immune system directly by moderately improving the number of immune cells that are capable of surveying for disease and destroying foreign pathogens. Structured Silver benefits the immune system indirectly by killing the bacteria and viruses that cause disease, thus reducing the workload of an already overworked immune system and allowing it to recharge.

Q: How long does Structured Silver stay in the body? Can it accumulate over time?
A: Research suggests that 98 percent of the Structured Silver leaves the body by the next day. Argyria can occur when the silver stays in the body, but you would have to drink a ten times normal dose for decades (and none of it could leave your body) before you would begin to have symptoms of argyria. It is the ionic and colloidal silver users that have too high concentrations of silver that cause argyria.

Suggested Resources

This booklet is not intended as a comprehensive text. For additional information, several resources are available.

Broader information about silver, how it works, scientific studies and additional applications can be found in other resources by Dr. Gordon Pedersen.

For information about a personal health issue, it is best to speak with your trusted health professional. This book cannot and is not intended to replace personalized care. Your doctor can be an excellent resource for improving your overall health – why not use them?

A broad introduction to the topic of silver in health can be found at the website of The Silver Health Institute: http://www.silverhealthinstitute.com.

To learn more about molecular structuring and structured water, an excellent primer comes in the form of a faculty lecture at the University of Washington by Dr. Gerald Pollack. This lecture, entitled "Water, Energy, and Life: Fresh Views from the Water's Edge" can be found at The Silver Health Institute's website. Further insight into the emerging research surrounding structured water is found in Dr. Pollack's newest book, "The Fourth Phase of Water."

For additional information and questions, many resources are available, including:

Acanlon E, et al. "Cost-effective faster wound healing with a sustained silver-releasing foam dressing in delayed healing leg ulcers – a health-economic analysis." Int Wound J. 2005 Jun; 2(2): 150-60.

Alexander, JW. "History of the Medical Use of Silver." Surg Infections 2009 Vol 10 No 3.

Berger TJ, et al. "Antifungal Properties of Electrically Generated Metallic Ions." Antimicrob Agents Chemother. 1976; (10): 856-60.

Bretana L, et al. "Antibacterial efficacy of a colloidal silver complex." Surg Forum. 1966; 17:76-8.

Chang AL, et al. "A case of argyria after colloidal silver ingestion." J Cutan Pathol. 2006 Dec;33(12):809-11.

Chang TW, Weinstein L. "Prevention of Herpes Keratoconjunctivitis in Rabbits by Silver Sulfadiazine." Antimicrob Agents Chemother. 1975; (80): 677-78.

Edwards-Jones V. "Antibacterial and barrier effects of silver against methicillin-resistant Staphylococcus aureus." J Wound Care. 2006 Jul; 15(7): 285-90.

Egger WA. "Antibiotic Resistance: Unnatural Selection in the Office and on the Farm." Wisconsin Medical Journal. Aug 2002.

Farber MP. "The Micro Silver Bullet." Houston. Professional Physician Publishing. 1995.

Fox CJ, 1968. "Silver sulfadiazine, a new topical therapy for Pseudomonas burns." Arch. Surg. 96:184-188.

Fox CJ, 1969. "Control of Pseudomonas infection in burns by Silver Sulfadiazine." Surg.Gynecol. Obstet. 128:1021-1026.

Hafkine A, 2003. "ASAP antiviral activity in Hepatitis B; DNA Polymerase Inhibition, Reverse Transcriptase Inhibition. Hafkine Institute for Training, Research and Testing.

Jurczak F, et al. "Randomized clinical trial of Hydrofiberdressing with silver versus povidone-iodine gauze in the management of open surgical and traumatic wounds." Int Wound J. 2007 Mar; 4(1): 66-76.

Paddock HN, et al. "A silver-impregnated antimicrobial dressing reduces hospital costs for pediatric burn patients." J Pediatr Surg. 2007 Jan;42(1): 211-3.

Powell J. "Silver: Our Mightiest Germ Fighter" Sci Digest. 1978; Mar 57-60.

Simonetti N, et al. "Electrochemical Ag+ for Preservative Use." Appl Enviro Microbial. 1992; (58): 3834-36.

Stoff J. "The Ultimate Nutrient." Tuscon. Insight Consulting Services. 2000.

Swartz MN. "Hospital acquired infections: diseases with increasingly limited therapies." Proc Noatl Acad Sci USA. 1994; 91(7): 2420-27.

Thurman R, Gerba C. "The Molecular Mechanisms of Copper and Silver Ion Disinfection of Bacteria and Viruses." CRC Crit Rev Envir Control. 1989; (18): 295-315.

Wenzel RP, Edmond MB. "The Impact of Hospital-Acquired Bloodstream Infections." Emerging Infectious Diseases. Vol. 7, No. 2. Mar-Apr 2001.

Zeller JL, et al. "JAMA patient page. MRSA infections." JAMA. 2007 Oct 17; 298(15): 1826.

Bibliography

1. http://www.davidsuzuki.org/issues/health/science/toxics/dir ty-dozen-cosmetic-chemicals/

2. Colloidal Silver: Medicinal Uses.

3. Carr, H., Wlodowski, T., 1973. Department of Microbiology, College of Physicians and Surgeons, Columbia University, New York, New York. Antimicrobial Agents and Chemotherapy. 10:585-587).

4. Clear Springs Press, Colloidal Silver.

5. Merck Manual of Diagnosis and Therapy, 1999 Section 226 (Toxic Nephropathy)

6. Merck Index., 1999. Silver. 1:645

7. IRIS Report, 2005.

8. EPA Report and Guidelines #D011.

9. http://www.atsdr.cdc.gov/toxfaqs/TF.asp?id=538&tid=97. April 10, 2013.

10. Pedersen, G., Indian Practitioner., 2010; 63(9);567-674. "Silver Sol completely removes Malaria parasites from the blood of human subjects infected with malaria in an average of five days: A review of four randomized, multi-centered, clinical studies performed in Africa."

Notes

Made in the USA
Charleston, SC
05 January 2015